Competition and Home Medicines

W. DUNCAN REEKIE

University of the Witwatersrand

and

HANS G. ÖTZBRUGGER

University of Innsbruck

Published by
THE INSTITUTE OF ECONOMIC AFFAIRS
1985

First published in May 1985

© THE INSTITUTE OF ECONOMIC AFFAIRS 1985

ISSN 0073-9103

ISBN 0-255 36181-5

Printed in Great Britain by
Goron Pro-Print Co. Ltd.,
Churchill Industrial Estate, Lancing, W. Sussex

Set in Univers 9 on 11pt Series 689

Contents

TABLES

FIGURES

Preface

IEA *Research Monographs* accommodate texts in which the emphasis is normally on the empirical content derived from documentary evidence, field studies, or other sources.

By chance, Research Monograph 39, *Competition and Home Medicines*, was written over a period of months during which the Secretary of State for Social Services, Mr Norman Fowler, was battling against considerable medical, industrial and political opposition to introduce a restricted list of drugs available for prescription on the National Health Service (NHS). His initiative reflected a concern shared by the authors of this *Monograph*, namely, that the NHS drugs bill has been rising rapidly—as have NHS expenditures generally. The proportion of NHS spending accounted for by drugs rose from 8·3 to 9·6 per cent between 1970 and 1984—which, against the background of fast-growing outlays on the NHS as a whole, amounted to an absolute increase of 5 per cent a year *in real terms*. Drugs now cost the NHS a total annual sum of £1,500 million.

Mr Fowler eventually got Parliamentary approval for a restricted list: from 1 April 1985 the brand-name products which doctors are permitted to prescribe on the NHS have been substantially reduced in seven therapeutic categories—tonics, antacids, laxatives, cough and cold remedies, vitamins, analgesics and tranquillisers—at an estimated saving to the public purse of £75 million a year. The final list is a much watered-down version of that which Mr Fowler originally proposed in November 1984 and which aimed to save £100 million annually. Largely as a result of intense lobbying by the doctors and the Association of the British Pharmaceutical Industry, the final list permits three times as many drugs as the November one. Moreover, even the forecast saving of £75 million may be optimistic. Other countries which have introduced similar restrictions on drugs (such as West Germany and Holland) have fallen well short of target savings because of a phenomenon known as 'diagnostic drift': doctors diagnose more

7

serious complaints to warrant more expensive drugs which remain available on prescription.

The authors of Research Monograph 39 are as disquieted as Mr Fowler by the rapidly-growing NHS drugs bill. And they are equally keen to encourage self-medication, within prudent safety limits, for relatively minor ailments so as to release NHS resources for more serious ones. Their approach, however, is different from his. Rather than removing doctors' freedom to prescribe, they argue that self-medication for minor ailments should be encouraged by measures which reduce the retail price and availability to consumers of home, or 'proprietary', medicines which can be sold over-the-counter without prescription. In other words, the more cheaply and easily increasingly prosperous consumers can purchase home medicines in retail outlets, the more they will choose to do so rather than troubling their doctor—thereby saving both their own time and their doctor's, and reducing NHS prescription costs.

Professor Reekie and Dr Ötzbrugger proceed from the empirical observation that people administer self-medication and use home medicines sensibly and responsibly. They choose intelligently between visiting a doctor and treating themselves. According to the authors, doctors claim that self-medication is successful in remedying complaints nine times out of 10.

With that re-assurance on the safety score, the authors identify what they perceive to be the principal constraint on home medicine sales (and indeed why home medicines are a declining sector of the UK pharmaceutical industry). It is, they argue, the virtually unique extent to which the industry is regulated in the Britain of 1985. While in some respects regulation can be said to be diminishing (more and more medicines which were formerly prescription-only have been re-classified for general or pharmacy-only sale), in other respects it has been on the increase. Restrictions on where, under what conditions, and in what quantity home medicines may be sold are now more stringent than ever, and the public advertising of certain products is no longer allowed. The Medicines Act of 1968, which subjected manufacturing of home medicines to a licensing procedure, has led to a significant number of producers leaving the industry and a consequent diminution of competition. And, last but not least, resale price maintenance (RPM) is alive and well and legal in home medicines, having been outlawed everywhere else many years ago.

The authors are in no doubt that excessive regulation of the home medicine industry harms consumers, producers, taxpayers, and specialised and other retailers of drugs who operate without a pharmacist on the premises. They also claim that the industry has considerable growth potential as more and more products are released from the prescription-only category—a development which can not only reduce the burden of the NHS on the taxpayer but also enlarge the role of the retail pharmacist in helping consumers select medicines which meet their requirements. In order that that potential can be realised, the authors make three principal recommendations: RPM in home medicines should be forbidden as a restrictive trade practice; the sale of more medicines in non-pharmacy outlets and a general freedom to advertise to consumers should be allowed; and the removal of drugs from prescription-only to over-the-counter sale should be speeded up.

The constitution of the Institute obliges it to dissociate its Trustees, Directors and Advisers from the analysis and conclusions of this *Research Monograph*. However, it offers the study as a thoughtful and well-reasoned contribution to helping alleviate the deep-seated conflict between the growing demand for health care and the reluctance of the taxpayer to finance the rapidly-rising expenditures of the NHS. Mr Fowler might usefully complement his 'black list' for drugs with a 'hit list' for de-regulation.

May 1985   Martin Wassell

The Authors

DR W DUNCAN REEKIE is E. P. Bradlow Professor of Business Economics at the University of the Witwatersrand, Johannesburg; previously Lecturer and subsequently Reader in Business Economics at the University of Edinburgh, 1969-83. Educated at the Universities of Edinburgh and Strathclyde, he has lectured widely in universities in New Zealand, Australia, Canada, Asia, the USA and Europe. He is a specialist in the economics of industrial organisation and has written several books on the pharmaceutical industry and on advertising. His writings have been published widely in the academic press, including *The Economic Journal, The Journal of Industrial Economics, Applied Economics, The Australian Economic Papers, The Scottish Journal of Political Economy,* and *The South African Journal of Economics.* He is the founder and editor of *Managerial and Decision Economics.* For the IEA he wrote Hobart Paper 79, *Give Us This Day...* (1978).

*　　*　　*

DR HANS G ÖTZBRUGGER is Lecturer in Economics at the University of Innsbruck. He received his MA in 1976 and his PhD in 1983 from that University.

Acknowledgements

We wish to thank Professor Bengt Jönsson of Linköping University, Sweden, Professor Sam Peltzman of the University of Chicago, USA, and Professor Michael Cooper of the University of Otago, New Zealand, for commenting on an early draft of this *Research Monograph.* Thanks are also due to Martin Wassell of the IEA for fastidious editing which undoubtedly improved the authors' style. Remaining faults can be attributed only to ourselves.

W.D.R.
H.G.O.

ONE

Introduction

This *Research Monograph* examines aspects of the regulation of competition in the home medicine or proprietary drug industry. The industry is almost unique in the Britain of 1985. It is subject to direct governmental control over price competition and promotional activity. It is also restricted by law in how and where it sells its products, and licences must be obtained before new products can be introduced to the market-place.

We shall argue that many of these restrictions on the competitive process serve the interests of certain professional, producing and retailing groups and not those of consumers as a whole. Furthermore, although there have been moves in recent years to liberalise some of the regulations controlling the industry, there have simultaneously been increases in the controls it is subject to. Given the contribution this industry can make to reducing the costs of conventional health care, one of the largest items of government expenditure, it is surprising that a Government allegedly pledged to cutting state spending should continue to hamper the activities of the industry. As we shall see, the industry can meet consumer wants in ways which are both economically and medically acceptable. That is to say, consumers, when permitted, are willing and able to pay for its products and do so spontaneously in the manner medical practitioners would recommend had they been independently consulted.

Defining the 'drug industry'

The 'drug industry', or pharmaceutical industry, can be defined extremely widely to include veterinary medicines, and on occasion even agrochemicals. We restrict ourselves here to medicines manufactured and sold for human use. That industry can be divided into two: the home medicine industry and the prescription pharmaceutical industry.[1] The definitional divide is not clear-cut

---

[1] The word 'ethical' refers to a subset of prescription medicines which must be advertised or promoted only to members of the medical, nursing or pharmacy professions.

since some medicines available over-the-counter (OTC) for purchase by the public cannot be publicly advertised. Others are available OTC, can be advertised to the medical profession, and can also be prescribed by doctors. At the extremes, many OTC medicines are never prescribed by doctors, while in the prescription medicine industry many can be advertised only to restricted professional groupings.

The two sectors also differ in other significant ways. Home medicines are essentially for relatively minor ailments such as transient headaches, aches or other pains, cuts, bruises, burns, coughs and colds. Prescription-only medicines are for more serious complaints, may be supplied only on a doctor's prescription, are not intended for self-treatment, and should be taken only with a physician's advice.

Product differentiation and research and development (R & D) to discover and develop new products for the market-place are important in both industries, but this importance differs in degree. In the prescription medicine industry, a high level of R & D is vital if a company is to survive. New products are frequently introduced; and if a company fails to improve the therapeutic qualities of efficacy and safety of the products in its range, it will rapidly lose market share to better-quality competitors. In the home medicine industry such competition by innovation is also present but is less intense. Typically, a product or brand has a longer life-cycle than does a prescription-only medicine.

Restrictions on distribution

Advertising of home medicines[1] is thus aimed mainly at the general public. The products are sold at low absolute monetary prices and at irregular but fairly frequent intervals. The nature of the advertising is, therefore, not dissimilar to that of most inexpensive, fast-moving consumer non-durables which are distributed through a variety of retail outlets. This statement must be

---

[1] Advertising and promotion of ethical medicines are directed not at consumers (patients) but at their agents (doctors). The degree of medical expertise possessed by the physician is considerably higher than that of the lay consumer of home medicines. Moreover, the products are both more potent and more liable to have side-effects. Thus, more specific and detailed data are required by the recipient of the medical advertising, and hence the nature of promotion tends to be relatively more educational and informative and more akin to that of advertising for industrial products rather than consumer goods. This difference in the style of the two types of medical promotion is further emphasised by the higher rate of product innovation in ethicals, and hence a further requirement to provide educational as opposed to reminder advertising.

modified slightly in that retail pharmacists are the traditional outlets for home medicines and offer advice to customers on a scale and of a quality not present in other channels of distribution used by the OTC industry (for example, grocery supermarkets and news-agents). Moreover, the distribution of certain types of home medicine has always been restricted to retail pharmacists. Since the Medicines Act of 1968, the products covered by such re-strictions have increased; and some products which are still available in non-pharmacy outlets (such as aspirin) cannot now be sold in such outlets in packs containing a larger than specified number of tablets or pills.

Price competition is also prohibited at the retail level. Indeed, home medicine is the only industry in Britain where resale price maintenance (or what Americans call 'fair trade' laws) survives.[1] The industry is thus heavily controlled in its overall marketing activities.

In the following sections, we first examine the home medicine industry in more detail, and then provide new information about the nature of the industry's marketing and competitive activities in the light of the regulatory framework. The concluding section summarises the role and importance of economic competition given the empirical evidence, and considers whether there should continue to be such strict regulation of both competition and marketing in the industry.

---

[1] Resale price maintenance (RPM) is the stipulation by the manufacturer of the price at which distributors may resell his product. A retailer providing the same services as competitors cannot undercut them in order to expand, nor can one providing fewer services charge correspondingly lower prices. This restrictive practice is prohibited by law in almost all British industries but it has been upheld as 'in the public interest' in home medicine. This contention is discussed at length in later pages. In the USA and Canada, price competition *is* permitted at the retail level. South Africa has the same prohibition as Britain.

TWO

The Home Medicine Industry

(a) Definitions

The industry supplies medicines which are available without prescription. They reach the public by over-the-counter (OTC) sale through a large number of retail outlets. The provisions of the Medicines Act restrict some to sale only if supervised by a pharmacist. Others are included in a General Sale List, and are widely available in corner shops, hotels and grocers, as well as in chemists' shops.

(b) The Responsible Consumer

It is well established that a state of total well-being is statistically abnormal. One typical study,[1] for example, recorded that 95 per cent of the people sampled reported some health complaints over the previous 14 days. In addition, the great majority of incidents of ill-health are managed by individuals themselves. The general types of complaints treated by the individual rather than the doctor have been categorised[2] as including worry, nervousness, headaches, coughs, colds and sore throats, back-aches, 'tummy troubles' and the like. These complaints are also the ailments regarded by doctors as suitable for self-medication.[3] Self-medication, in short, appears to be applied sensibly and responsibly by most consumers; it is used not as an alternative to medical consultation but rather as a complement when appropriate.[4] The argument that the industry must be regulated because

---

[1] M. E. J. Wadsworth, W. H. J. Butterfield, and R. Blaney, *Health and Sickness: the Choice of Treatment*, Tavistock, 1971.

[2] D. C. Morrell and C. J. Wale, 'Symptoms perceived and recorded by patients', *Journal of the Royal College of General Practitioners*, 1976; J. H. F. Brotherston, in J. Pemberton and H. Willard (eds.), *Recent Studies in Epidemiology*, Oxford University Press, 1958.

[3] Office of Health Economics, *Without Prescription*, OHE, 1968.

[4] N. Kessel and D. M. Shepherd, 'The health and attitudes of people who seldom consult a doctor', *Medical Care*, 1965.

consumers would not otherwise act in their own best interests appears to be weak.

(c) The Shifting Costs of Health Care

The corollary is that

'the availability of such medicines . . .reduces the calls on doctors and assists them in deploying their skills to the best advantage. The NHS (National Health Service) would be quite unable to deal with the extra demand which would be unleashed in the absence of medicines available for sale over the counter'.[1]

This is a major benefit to the state at a time when rising costs of health care are a significant cause of concern. This is true not only in the UK, with its NHS, but throughout the world. The costs of health care are rising as expectations of what is 'good health' increase, and as technology advances and more expensive forms of treatment become available. All nations are expressing concern about these developments, whether the method of providing health care is primarily through the state or by private insurance. In the USA, the increasing use of Medicare and Medicaid, by the elderly and indigent respectively, is straining governmental budgets. In Germany, where the provision of health care is primarily by contributions from employers and employees to private social security schemes, government is also concerned since ever-increasing deductions from the wages of employees have resulted directly in a reduction in the government's tax base and, indirectly, in trade union pressure on government to 'do something'.

If self-medication can be used to shift the costs of medical care from third-party reimbursement schemes (state or private), it will release both monetary and real resources which can then be redirected towards more acute conditions.

(d) An Industry in Transition?

Health services vary among countries. For this reason (and because of international price differences), consumer expenditure on OTC drugs varies immensely. Of the countries in Table 1, expenditure in the UK is the lowest, with the average French household spending 20 times as much.

Nor is this a statistical abnormality for one year only. The British home medicine industry is smaller as a proportion of population

---

[1] The Price Commission, *Prices, Costs and Margins in the Production and Distribution of Proprietary Non-ethical Medicines*, HC 469, HMSO, 1978, para. 2.4.

than that of most other developed countries; and it has reached this position after several years of relative decline. The home medicine industry shrank from 15 to 13 per cent of total pharmaceutical output (measured at manufacturers' selling prices) between 1970 and 1981.[1]

The retail income of pharmacies, since 1971, shows a similar picture. The total turnover of chemists' shops (at retail prices) rose by 50 per cent in the 1960s, and then doubled by the mid-1970s. Non-NHS sales (including home medicines) rose by 40 per cent in the 1960s and grew only one-third as fast as NHS sales in the 1970s. In consequence, non-NHS sales through chemists' shops had fallen to around one-third of total sales in 1981, compared with around two-thirds in 1961.[2]

Thus the UK home medicine industry is a declining sector of the pharmaceutical industry. One possible cause of this decline in an industry which, in total, is regarded as a growth sector may

Table 1:
Household Expenditure on Pharmaceuticals:
Selected Countries, 1977
(*In US dollars at retail prices*)

	Per household	% of total retail sales
Australia	227	3·2
Austria	35	0·7
Belgium	250	3·7
Denmark	80	1·0
Finland	190	3·7
France	399	5·0
Germany	83	1·5
Italy	149	4·0
Netherlands	119	1·5
New Zealand	81	1·0
Norway	81	1·1
Spain	86	2·0
Sweden	201	2·5
Switzerland	119	1·4
UK	20	0·5
USA	187	1·9

Source: Euromonitor, London. Estimates are based on family expenditure data.

[1] Association of the British Pharmaceutical Industry (ABPI) (annual reports).
[2] *Nielsen Researcher* (various years).

be the continuously growing use of the NHS by the public. The number of prescriptions dispensed rose by 24 per cent between 1970 and 1980, from 306 to 374 million. In 1980, the average cost to the NHS of each prescription was £2·37. Only 25 per cent of prescriptions were subject to the flat-rate charge of £1·40, the remainder being dispensed to people exempted from it. Eighty-eight million prescriptions, 24 per cent of the 1979 total, were for drugs affecting the central nervous system. Between 1966 and 1975, prescriptions for anti-depressants more than doubled from 4·2 to 9·1 million. Prescriptions for tranquillisers rose to 24·3 million. Industry spokesmen see this rise in prescriptions for tranquillisers as one of the causes of the decline in consumption of analgesics (that is, aspirins and paracetamols), a major segment of the home medicine market.[1]

A second factor which cannot have improved the commercial health of the industry is the absolute decline in the number of retail chemists. The number of pharmacies in Britain has fallen steadily over the years—from 14,620 in 1962 to 10,711 in 1981.[2] A third source of the commercial malaise may lie in the more stringent governmental rules and regulations of the last few years which have raised the industry's costs while squeezing its revenues.[3]

(e) The Threat to the Independent Retailer

The independent retailer is becoming ever more dependent on prescription medicines for his turnover. His other traditional products of the 1950s and earlier (such as cameras and cosmetics) are now sold more efficiently in other specialised outlets (using the word 'efficiently' to indicate compliance with consumer preferences). The same is not true of the multiple pharmacists, such as Boots, which have retained their share of sales in such product groups, and indeed have diversified still further away from the products of the apothecary.

Not only is the independent pharmacist under commercial threat from other retailers; he is also being challenged from within his own profession by multiple chain pharmacies. UK data are

---

[1] Proprietary Association of Great Britain (PAGB) in written evidence to the Price Commission: *Prices, Costs and Margins in the Production and Distribution of Proprietary Non-ethical Medicines*, HC 469, HMSO, London, 1978.

[2] *The Pharmaceutical Register*, various years.

[3] W. D. Reekie, 'Legislative Change and Industrial Performance: A Case Study', *Scottish Journal of Political Economy*, 1980.

difficult to obtain; in the USA, as Table 2 indicates, the multiple chain was responsible for one-fifth of the dispensing in 1974 but only a little under one-third by 1983. Indeed, between 1982 and 1983, chains increased the amount of prescriptions they dispensed by 7 per cent, compared with only 0·5 per cent for the independents. As in the UK, the independents rely much more on prescription than on non-prescription sales (57·9 per cent of total store business against 15·1 per cent). And again, as in the UK, their reliance on what is effectively a statutory monopoly is increasing.

Table 2:
Multiple Chains as a Percentage of
Total Prescriptions: USA, 1974 to 1983

	Volume %	Value %
1974	21·7	21·3
1978	24·6	25·1
1980	26·8	26·5
1982	28·7	28·9
1983	30·1	30·3

Source: American Druggist, May 1984, p. 14.

In the USA, price competition at the pharmacy level is permitted (for both ethical and OTC drugs). This contrasts with, for example, the UK, Germany and South Africa where RPM is still upheld. In consequence, the US independent faces additional pressure as American state and private health insurance schemes attempt to curb health care expenditures. This was amplified as follows in a recent article in the American Druggist:

'Among developments that could create third-party trouble for many pharmacies is the relatively new cost-containment mechanism known as the "preferred provider organisation" (PPO). Pioneered by private health insurers, usually in response to pressure from employers, this approach is now being looked at by Medicaid also. A PPO is a group of providers who agree to provide services at a discount to an insurer's beneficiaries, in return for the insurer's agreement to channel the beneficiaries to them. While the concept was originally applied to physician and dentist services, insurance companies have begun extending it to pharmaceutical services. The only way a pharmacist can avoid losing business when a PPO shows up is to join it'.[1]

---

[1] American Druggist, May 1984, p. 18.

Chains will generally be in a better financial position to accept the lower selling prices implied, partly because of their stronger bargaining power when buying and partly because they can practice price discrimination across a diversified range of products in their stores in a way the much more specialised independent cannot.

(f) Industry Structure

A major problem in analysing the home medicine industry is, as we have already seen, one of definition. There is an ethical convention in the medical profession that home medicines advertised publicly should not be prescribed by doctors, and in practice they rarely are. Conversely, many home medicines have never been publicly advertised but come to the consumer's notice through frequent prescription and recommendation by doctors (Panadol, Senokot, Benylin, for example). A further difficulty is that the market is sub-divided into therapeutic groups with a high cross-elasticity of supply. Sub-markets exist for analgesics, cough and cold remedies, indigestion remedies, laxatives, germicides and antiseptics, and eye-care preparations. The problem is not insurmountable, particularly if we could be sure that the cross-elasticity of demand between these groups was low. But this is not always the case. Products such as effervescent analgesics are frequently used as laxatives as well as for headaches. And recent years have seen the introduction of night cold remedies and medicated lemon drinks—Night Nurse and Lemsip, for example—in the cough and cold market which have further eroded the consumer's reliance on non-combination analgesics.

Using an Instability Index

As measured by market structure, the sub-markets are not highly concentrated (that is, a small number of products does *not* account for the bulk of sales). Table 3 gives data on concentration which support this contention and which, by comparing pairs of years, also show how competitive some of the various markets are in terms of product rivalry. The modified Hymer-Pashigian Instability Index is used in the Table because markets can undergo changes of economic importance which are not revealed in concentration ratios. For example, the firms making up the concentration ratio may change in relative importance; only the top firms are considered, and even they may not be the same in two different periods.[1] In addition, the other disregarded firms or brands may also alter in competitive importance. The Index used here employed the formula:

$$\sum_{i=1}^{n} \left(S_{i,\ 1982} - S_{i,\ 1973} \right)$$

where n equals the number of brands (generally, there is only one brand for each firm) and S equals the market share of the ith firm in 1982 or 1973. The algebraic signs of the market-share changes were ignored. Thus the Hymer-Pashigian Index takes account of all firms in the market but is little affected by the movements of small ones, or by small movements by large firms. Consequently, the higher its value, the more 'competitive' the market is in terms of a lack of prolonged market dominance.[2]

The Instability Index also overcomes the defects of the Spearman rank correlation coefficient[3] as an index of 'competition by mobility'. Let us consider two duopolies (that is, two-firm markets, or markets with only two sellers) in periods t and t+1. In one instance, the firms may move from market shares of 90 per cent and 10 per cent respectively to 60 and 40 per cent. The rank correlation would be unity (positive), indicating no competition, while the Instability Index would take on a value of 60·0. In the second instance, the firms may simply reverse their market shares of 51 and 49 per cent. Then the rank correlation coefficient would, at unity (negative), indicate maximum competitive mobility, but the Instability Index would register only the low value of 4·0.

The values achieved in Table 3 are well above the maximum which Hymer and Pashigian observed in their original study of American industries, which indicates that the 'top is a very slippery place' in home medicines. Moreover, since the Index was calculated across sub-markets and not for the industry as a whole,

---

[1] The 'concentration ratio' is a technical term denoting the percentage of industry sales (or some other variable) held by the leading brands or firms in the market.

[2] S. Hymer, and P. Pashigian, 'Turnover of firms as a measure of market behaviour', *Review of Economics and Statistics*, 1962.

[3] 'Rank correlation' is a statistical construct which can be readily understood by reference to sporting league tables. For example, if in a four-team football league, Clubs W, X, Y and Z are ranked at the end of two successive seasons in the order just listed, the coefficient is (plus) 1·0. If, however, the order is totally reversed in the second season, to Z, Y, X, W, the coefficient is (minus) 1·0. The calculated value can be anywhere between these two extremes. A value of (minus) 1·0 indicates 'perfect' team mobility, and of (plus) 1·0 'perfect' stability.

Table 3:
Sub-markets and Measures of Concentration
in the Home Medicine Industry, 1973 and 1982

	Market size (1982) (millions of users)	3-Product Ratios 1973	3-Product Ratios 1982	Hymer-Pashigian Index
Mouthwash, gargles and remedies for mouth ulcers	18·3	72·8	55·7	95·0
Cough mixtures	23·6	52·3	54·3	128·0
Throat lozenges and pastilles	23·1	49·0	34·5	98·4
Cold and 'flu remedies	27·6	46·9	41·4	91·6
Headache remedies and analgesics	34·7	44·2	41·1	43·8
Eye lotions and ointments	11·9	90·5	84·1	22·8
Indigestion and stomach remedies	20·0	53·6	46·1	45·0
Rubs and rheumatism remedies	13·5	54·7	61·7	34·4
Haemorrhoid and piles remedies	5·9	n.a.	60·1	n.a.
Vitamin tablets and capsules	9·9	68·4	53·2	40·1
Tonics	5·6	52·0	56·5	34·2
Laxatives and salts	12·3	69·0	68·4	18·0
Ointments and salves	30·9	71·3	65·6	31·1

Source: Authors' calculations using recall data from the *Target Group Index* published by the British Market Research Bureau. Market size is given in millions of the adult population of the UK who had suffered from the defined complaint at least once in the year prior to the sample interview (i.e , 1982).

the values may be more significant than any obtained for highly aggregated but economically unrelated industry groups. As can also be seen, the ratios tend to have fallen where the sub-markets were highly concentrated. Moreover, it can be inferred from the consistently high Instability Indices either that consumers are very disloyal to brands or that new brands are frequently entering the markets and, ultimately, some are gaining consumer acceptance. It is the undisputed opinion of most members of the industry and of outside observers that there is 'strong brand loyalty'.[1] This supports the latter rather than the former explanation, namely, that product innovation is frequent and on occasion successful

---

[1] The Price Commission, 1978, *op. cit.*, para. 5.21.

in most of the markets specified in the Table. (For analgesics, part of the explanation is also the shift away from aspirin towards paracetamol, in both the branded and own-brand sectors.)

In the cold remedy market, Lemsip, Medinite, and Night Nurse—products which soothe coughs, subdue cold symptoms and also aid sleep—have tended to displace the more traditional products such as Beecham's Powders. In cough medicines, the major advance (between 1973 and 1982, Table 3) has been Benylin, an unadvertised product which has grown from a near-14 per cent share to control over a third of the segment. In laxatives, also, it is an unadvertised product which has performed most spectacularly. Senokot has grown from a 17 to a 28 per cent share of the market. Clearly, word-of-mouth recommendation by doctor, pharmacist or friend is a most effective form of promotion in the home medicine industry.

(g) The Industry and Government

Three main governmental Reports or Acts have had an impact on the British industry in recent years: the National Board for Prices and Incomes' Report of 1968,[1] the Medicines Act of the same year, and the Price Commission's Report of 1978. The last two have had by far the most profound influence.

Promotion, choice and costs

The NBPI Report took the view that advertising in the home medicine industry is necessary either *per se* or as an alternative to the efforts at the retail stage of the pharmacist or other shop-keeper. Table 4 illustrates how manufacturers' expenditures on advertising and other forms of sales promotion are to some extent a substitute for the retail margins which would otherwise be required to compensate the retailer for lower turnover and en-hanced risk in selling a less heavily advertised product. Paragraph 60 of the NBPI Report stated that

'with proprietary medicines promoted with a view to direct purchase by the public, the usual practice . . . is to allow the retailer a percentage of the retail price . . . designed to reflect the selling effort required'.

In an innovative environment with a high degree of consumer choice, this inducement is inevitable.

---

[1] National Board for Prices and Incomes, *Distributors' margins on Paint, Children's Clothing, Household Textiles and Proprietary Medicines*, Cmnd. 3737, HMSO, London, 1968.

Table 4:
Basic Margins Available on Proprietary Medicines

	Before Purchase Tax (per cent of retail selling price)	After Purchase Tax (per cent of retail selling price)
Nationally advertised, fast-moving brands of leading manufacturers	18–25	15–20
Unadvertised, slow-moving products	25–33½	20–27

Source: National Board for Prices and Incomes, 1968, *op. cit.*, para. 70.

To quote Professor Israel Kirzner:

'[The businessman has] not only to produce opportunities which are available to consumers; [he has] to make consumers aware of these opportunities. . . . An affluent society is one in which there are many, many opportunities placed before the consumer . . . and if he is to make a sensible decision he is going to have to spend several hours calculating very carefully, reading, re-reading everything that's on the packages. . . . It's a tough job to be a consumer. And the multiplicity of opportunities makes it necessary for advertisers, for producers, to project more and more provocative messages if they want to be heard. This is the cost of affluence. It is a cost, certainly; something that we'd much rather do without, if we could; but we can't'.[1]

In short, choice is difficult and costly for consumers (either because of the time they spend on searching or because of the mental stress of decision-making). Advertising and retail displays cut that cost but do not eliminate it. Outside of Nirvana, nothing can reduce transaction costs to zero. Policy-makers, therefore, should direct their attention to the least-cost method of assisting consumers to make choices.

Are profits 'unreasonable'?

If advertising is a necessary cost in an affluent society, and if a simple, unadorned statement giving information about a product will simply not be noticed; if the role of the manufacturer's salesmen, and the counter worker helping to 'push' goods through the distribution channel has been superseded by manufacturers' advertising directed at the consumer—who in turn demands of distributors that they stock the desired brand and so 'pull' goods through the channel—can we take the next step in the chain of analysis and argue that this 'necessary' cost of advertising is the least costly, most efficient alternative?

---

[1] I. Kirzner, 'Advertising', *The Freeman*, 1972.

We can if the industry is deemed competitive—that is, if prices and profits can be considered 'fair'. 'Fairness' is a word with no objective meaning. 'Unfair' monopoly power exists if a firm or industry can *persistently* earn higher profits, charge higher prices, or run itself in an inefficient manner. The only yardstick for identifying this ability *persistently* to act monopolistically is the presence or absence of entry barriers to the industry—not prices, profits or marketing expenditures themselves. In isolation, the latter data tell us nothing. If, however, prices or profits *could* be lower, and if marketing costs *could* be reduced, then entrant firms will appear and charge lower prices, operate at a lower cost, and in turn earn (temporarily) higher profits than they otherwise could. Are there barriers to entry in home medicines? This is the key question.

The threat of entry into the UK's home medicine industry must be considered high, given the large number of manufacturers of *prescription* medicines who employ salesmen who often visit the same retail outlets (that is, pharmacists). If *proprietary* medicine firms are earning profits which are 'unreasonable', entry would be expected to occur promptly by, for example, established ethical firms with the assistance of their undoubted advertising expertise. That such entry rarely occurs puts the onus of proof on those who assert that the industry's profits are 'excessive' in some way.

The Price Commission, which succeeded the NBPI in 1973 (after an interval of four years), took a different view of advertising. In several instances,[1] it claimed (without empirical evidence) that advertising had raised prices, with consequential 'unreasonable' profits. The Commission tended not to produce the type of information which would help understanding of the role of advertising in the competitive process, as the NBPI did. This may have been due to bias or to changes in marketing conditions between the 1960s and 1970s.

The issue, however, is not really *company profitability* but *individual product contribution* to profits. Again, however, the question is begged why entry does not occur in those therapeutic sectors where product contribution is high.[2] (The products

---

[1] W. D. Reekie, *Advertising and Price*, The Advertising Association, 1979.

[2] 'Contribution' is an accounting term defined as 'sales less fixed costs' where fixed costs include advertising, R & D and other overhead expenditure. Some products may be priced so as simply to cover their variable costs of production and distribution, in which case contribution to overheads and profits is close to zero. In others, price may be well above average variable costs, in which case the average contribution is high.

singled out for attack in the Price Commission's Report were Anadin, Disprin, Milk of Magnesia, Rennies, Beecham's Powders, and Optrex eye lotions.) The reason cannot be that there are manufacturing, advertising or other promotional barriers to entry. As we have already noted, there are several dozen prescription medicine firms already operating in Britain with the requisite expertise in each of these fields. Any one of them could readily enter such markets if profits were 'abnormally attractive'.

One possible clue to why they do not is that the industry's average return on capital is around 20 per cent on an 'historic cost' basis[1]— which is not far above that of manufacturing industry generally. In short, *within firms* a considerable degree of *variation in the contribution of different products* must exist. This being so, it would be relatively easy for existing firms dramatically to reduce the price of a high-contribution product and raise comparatively slightly the prices of others which contribute less. Such a step could go some way towards maintaining overall profitability whilst simultaneously deterring entry into specific fields. Entrants would then be attracted only if the average profitability of firms was 'excessively high' so that no reshuffling of contributions and prices could maintain the original average.[2]

In short, one reason why entry does not occur is probably because such a re-jigging of contributions and prices may be unnecessary since the present price structure may already be optimal, given differences in the price sensitivities and product preferences of consumers, and in the cost structures of products. If so, any adjustment would reduce the average profits of companies (and *exit* rather than entry would occur). These conclusions were supported, if not confirmed, in the Price Commission's Report:

'Contributions are often quite high and are being used . . . to develop and launch new products—often a costly business' (p. 3, para. 17);
'A spectrum of contributions . . . from low to high is therefore not unexpected' (para. 4.7).

In view of these arguments, it is surprising that the Commission was 'disturbed' at this finding (para. 4.7). *The Times* reported on 19 May 1978 that 'In one of its hardest hitting reports yet, the Price Commission has criticised patent medicine manufacturers

---

[1] The Price Commission, 1978, *op. cit.*, p. 3, para. 15.

[2] Professor Sam Peltzman of the University of Chicago has pointed out to us that an additional reason for the 'high' profitability is the high product turnover (Table 3) and high company exit (Table 5): 'The losses of unsuccessful firms which have exited are not being counted'. (Correspondence with Professor Peltzman.)

for charging too much' and also, said *The Guardian* on the same day, 'for high profit margins and large amounts spent on advertising'. Nonetheless, 'disturbed' it was, not only by the variability of the contributions which different products made to profits but also by the variability in ratios of advertising to sales:

'The fact that some manufacturers maintain [relatively low advertising] puts into question the ratios at the top of the range' (p. 4, para. 21),

and

'such high levels of margins and the cost to consumers of such high levels of advertising are matters which would be justified only in *exceptional* circumstances' (para. 9.4—emphasis added).

What is so naive in these statements about above-average advertising and contributions to profits is their failure to mention that an average is only the approximate mid-point of a range. By definition, about half of all data on profits or advertising will be below the average and the other half above it. In itself, an average carries very little meaning. The spread between the lowest and highest figures is also relevant. That depends on conditions of both demand and supply. On the supply side, the Commission notes, despite its conclusions, that a new product *'may incur a loss for a few years* before it becomes established; introduction . . . takes several years and *is expensive'* (para. 4.7—emphasis added). Advertising in turn, of new products must be 'disproportionate for a lengthy period . . . about five years' (para. 5.3). On the demand side, as well as increasing brand throughput, advertising can 'enhance the [generally accepted] benefit [of the medicine resulting from] psychological factors' (para. 5.5).

In brief, for a firm to make adequate profits from its product range it must cross-subsidise the products. New products must be subsidised by older ones with low overheads but a large potential for economies of scale and rapidly occurring break-even points. The higher the output required to break even or to attain economies of scale, the larger the advertising volume required—even for older products.[1]

Competition by place of sale

Another factor influencing rivalry among firms is that not all home medicines are sold through the same distribution channels. Some

---

[1] This explains the Commission's puzzlement that some firms 'spend much more [on advertising than others] even on established products. *Therefore* . . . advertising is excessive'. (Price Commission, 1978, *op. cit*, para. 5.24—emphasis added).

are on the 'General Sale List' of the Medicines Act and can be sold in any retail outlet. Others, however—anti-histamines, vaso-constrictors, and codeine products, for example—are permitted to be sold only under the personal supervision of a pharmacist, implying not only a limitation to pharmacy-only sale but also a restriction on the display methods which can be used. Other things equal, innovations in the latter product category will take much longer to achieve a break-even volume than those in the former.[1] The volume of advertising required to reach 55 million potential consumers is, however, identical. It thus becomes probable that advertising to sales ratios will be higher for pharmacy-only products than for those on the General Sale List. It does not follow that some advertising is excessive but simply that its volume is necessary to provide the required profit and sales figures, given the relevant technology of distribution. For reasons of timing, availability of capital, changes in consumer tastes, production methods or whatever, the firm's entrepreneurial judgement is that advertising is the best way to help satisfy consumer demand.

For anyone to suggest after the event that advertising is not the correct way to satisfy consumer wishes is to claim for himself powers of omniscience. Snapshot views of any market rarely provide significant pictures of the competitive whole.

Different products manufactured by the same firm can have widely differing rates of profitability, levels of contribution, and advertising to sales ratios. In industries such as proprietary medicines, these variations within firms are inevitable and no inferences can be drawn about a positive relationship between entry barriers and advertising. Indeed, the reverse is true. In proprietary medicines, entry is relatively easy, potential entrants abound, and, as entry theory predicts, the profitability of the industry is close to the average return on capital in manufacturing industry—which suggests neither a shortage nor excess of funds in the industry and implies nothing by way of monopoly profits 'protected' by the 'barriers' of advertising.

It is certainly arguable that the Price Commission should be heavily criticised for misjudging the meaning and strength of competition in the industry. On the other hand, the Commission was also seriously hampered by its terms of reference, which precluded it explicitly from examining the totality of the market and so severely limited the area within which competition could be presumed to exist.

---

[1] There are about 10,000 pharmacists, but over 110,000 retailers, including pharmacies, who can and do sell home medicines.

Any misjudgement by the Commission of the threat of potential competition, or an inability to specify it, was a direct result of the limits within which it had to work. For example, and ignoring the prescription medicine producers, the Commission was restricted to examining medicines available for sale over the counter to the general public. It was, however, precluded from examining those medicines (around 900) which *were* available OTC but which were advertised only to the medical profession, even though they could be obtained without prescription.

In addition, the Commission's terms of reference also prevented it from studying another 1,200 products which were available to the general public OTC but received no advertising back-up at all. In total, something in the region of 2,100 products could not be examined by the Commission; its pronouncements were restricted to findings derived from a sample of 90 or so of the 300 products it was allowed to investigate which were manufactured by 36 firms or divisions of firms.[1]

No outside agency, however erudite, can be a substitute for a market test of competition. But it is at least incumbent on a body such as the Price Commission, whose general remit was to strengthen competitive market forces, to examine the market in its totality. Or, if specific instructions forbade this course, strong protests should have been made against such limitations (rather than mild acceptance of them).

Since the enactment of the Medicines Act of 1968, there has been widespread exit from the industry. Manufacture is now subject to the issue of licences. As the Commission reported in 1978:

'The standards required to satisfy the licensing authorities have led to some companies discontinuing a variety of products and even to abandon manufacture altogether'.[2]

Controls are imposed on handling and manufacturing facilities, staff qualifications, description of goods, claims and labelling. Costs have been raised, and the wealthier consumer who can afford and is prepared to buy from the higher-cost manufacturer is duly protected. The higher-cost manufacturer is in turn protected from the low-cost producer who previously had sold to more price-sensitive consumers. Table 5 shows how legislation has encouraged exit from the industry and so diminished competition— a process which is likely to continue.

---

[1] The Price Commission, 1978, *op. cit.*, p. 1, para. 2 and para. 1.4.

[2] The Price Commission, 1978, *op. cit.*, para. 28.

Table 5:
Effects of the 1968 Medicines Act on Generic (Unbranded) and Non-ethical Products (advertising not restricted to medical profession)

	Non-ethical producers	Generic producers
Sample of firms	26	10
Extra staff employed on quality control (number and %)	107 (26%)	54 (30%)
Number of generics phased out due to the Act	30	472
Number of non-ethicals phased out due to the Act	79	19

Note: Product licences also add to current costs since part of the licence fee is related to turnover (0·25 to 0·5 per cent).

Source: The Price Commission, 1978, *op. cit.*, para. 2.9.

As the Price Commission observed:

'The number of proprietary non-ethical medicines is likely to diminish substantially as the impact of the Act continues to spread. Those disappearing are likely to be the lesser-known ones with small local sales, rather than those nationally advertised, which are more likely to meet the standards of the licensing authority. Manufacturers of these products . . . are finding difficulty in meeting the cost of the quality standards'. (para. 2.12)

The Commission merely uttered these remarks; it made no attempt to evaluate their impact on competition. If they were valid, entry theory would predict that competitive forces would be diminished. The question remains begging why a body whose remit included the promotion of competition passed no judgement on the anti-competitive outcome of the Medicines Act.

Competition by price

The Commission was also expressly forbidden from commenting on the practice of RPM in pharmaceuticals (above, p. 13). RPM is permitted in home medicines as a consequence of a judgement of the Restrictive Trade Practices Court that retailers must not sell home medicines below the manufacturers' recommended retail price. This protects the gross margin of the retailer, and in particular of the retail pharmacist. The argument for protection is that the skills of the pharmacist are of great value to the community; if pharmacists had to compete on price with other retail outlets, such as multiple grocers, their numbers would decline and the community would be deprived of their expertise.[1]

The Commission was not prohibited, however, from commenting on the reluctance of retail pharmacists to exploit the differentials in manufacturers' recommended prices between identical or similar medicaments.[2] However, it merely noted that the 'professional ethics of the pharmacist forbid price competition by means of point-of-sale promotion' (para. 3.8). Why did the Commission not condemn this as a restrictive practice which inhibits entry to the industry by lower-priced manufacturers unable or unwilling to advertise? There is evidence that point-of-sale advertising lowers consumer prices, and the Commission itself maintained that it would be in the interests of the consumer for competition to be furthered by more information about (non-advertised) products being made available (para. 9.10). The Commission did not suggest how this last recommendation should be implemented. It is a pity that the 'professional ethics' and skills of the pharmacist should have been confused with 'restrictive practices'. The two are distinct, and the Commission should have tried to foster the first (in the consumer's interest) whilst weakening or destroying the second (also for the sake of the consumer).

'Professional ethics' is a phrase frequently used to justify a restrictive practice. The practice defended is alleged to be 'in the public interest' but on closer scrutiny it often seems to be operating against the best interest of consumers and the prime beneficiaries are instead the existing professional group which strives to defend it. A parallel can be drawn with the recent removal of the monopoly of opticians over the sale of spectacles, which has resulted in an in-store display of the prices of spectacle frames on a scale hitherto unknown. The relaxation of regulation has produced more

---

[1] Sometimes RPM is also defended on the ground that it exists to discourage over-use of medicines merely because they are price-promoted. This argument is implausible. A person suffering from a headache, for example, is unlikely to consume simultaneously four aspirins instead of two because the price of the package was lower. In practice, once the package has been paid for, the monetary cost to the consumer of increasing his dose from two to four would be zero. Consumers of medicines, however, do not behave in such an irresponsible fashion. Neither is it plausible to move from simultaneous extra consumption to extra consumption due to prolonged and continuous self-medication, say, of a laxative, after the consumer perceives he is cured.

[2] While it is true that RPM ensures there is no price competition between retail outlets on a particular brand, there is significant competition between brands. There are *at least* three discernible price levels. In hot lemon cold products, for example, the brand leader, Lemsip, is the most expensive, Hot Lemon is priced below Lemsip, and the own-label brands, e.g. Boots, Superdrug, etc., are priced at the lowest level.

price competition accompanied by in-store promotion.

The recent UK Office of Fair Trading report on *Opticians and Competition* explained why this was so and stated that:

'the advertising restrictions result in prices being significantly higher and efficiency significantly lower than they otherwise would be. . . .

The Rules on Publicity 1981 effectively deny consumers information on available opticians in their locality, the range and prices of available products, the services which are offered by opticians in terms of opening hours, speed of dispensing, product guarantees and specialised services such as contact lens work, and, to a lesser extent, quality. Consumers are therefore denied the knowledge on which to make an informed choice of optician.

This lack of knowledge on the part of consumers has the effect of increasing the ability of opticians to fix prices without regard to the prices of other opticians and thereby to recover their overheads while operating below capacity. . . .

. . . the Rules on Publicity make it more difficult for new firms to enter the market and . . . [the Rules] may act as a disincentive to innovation.

We have examined the opticians' assertion that advertising would lead to a general reduction in the quality of prescribing and dispensing and of the eye examination, and such direct evidence as is available, notably the study by the Federal Trade Commission. We find no basis for the opticians' fears'.[1]

In essence, most consumers of spectacles are long-sighted and can select their own lenses whilst reading a printed page without an optician's assistance. Those consumers who are short-sighted will, as they always have done, tend to use an optician for eye testing where the problem of lens selection for distant vision is more complex. In either event, the removal of a 'professional restriction' was found by the OFT to be in the consumer's interest.

It may not, however, be quite so easy to implement this type of legislative repeal with home medicines where regulation has become more, not less, stringent. Since August 1978, the promotion of certain medicines, and treatments for certain types of disease, have no longer been permitted in publicly-circulated journals.[2] The list of medicines restricted to retail sale by pharmacists (that is, outlets registered by the Pharmaceutical Society) has increased since that date, and the maximum pack-sizes for many analgesics sold by non-pharmacists has now been restricted to 25 tablets or 10 powders.[3] Such changes 'in the availability of large pack-sizes . . . are significantly eroding . . . price differential(s)'.[4] In short, as Table 5 indicates, the manufacturing

---

[1] Office of Fair Trading report, *Opticians and Competition*, HMSO, 1983, pp. 140-141.

[2] The Price Commission, 1978, *op. cit.*, para. 2.9.

[3] *Ibid.*, para. 2.11.   [4] *Ibid.*, para. 2.12.

economies which many small-scale firms with low promotion budgets can obtain by packaging in large containers for concentrated (local) distribution have been eroded, and cost advantages gained by large-scale national distributors with national promotion budgets who typically sell at a premium price. The result can only have been a diminution of competition in the industry. Although the facts (Table 5) were remarked on, not a word of condemnation of these regulatory changes was apparent in the Price Commission's Report. Yet the changes have resulted in entry barriers which are not in the consumer's interest.

THREE

Competition in Home Medicines

(a) The Market

Before a product can be brought to the market, it is necessary to know who has a demand for it and therefore requires information about it. Figure 1 helps answer this question for home medicines. In the year ending 31 March 1982, a sample of 24,000 adults (aged 15 and over) representing the population of Great Britain was asked: 'Have you suffered from this complaint in the last 12 months?'. The question referred to eight illnesses. In the Figure the responses are categorised by age groups.

The Figure highlights how the ailments are distributed as a proportion of the relevant *total* age group at risk. For six diseases (coughs, sore throats, colds, 'flu, headaches and hayfever), the younger age groups are more obviously at risk than the older. Only with arthritis and rheumatism is the reverse clearly true. In general, people become less prone to a disease after the age of 25.

The graphs in Figure 1 could thus imply (except for diseases related specifically to the ageing process, such as rheumatism and arthritis) that younger people are more susceptible to illness than older ones; and that as people become older their immunity to illness grows. An equally valid interpretation would be that the community standard of what is considered 'good health' is rising and that it is the younger members of society who are expressing most strongly this change in demand or preference for complete physical well-being. What was tolerated in previous decades or by older people today as 'normal', or as a minor physical nuisance, is now regarded as a medically unacceptable condition and is registered as a complaint.[1]

(b) Product Usage

We noted in Section 2 that most home medicines are bought

---

[1] This theory has been more fully developed by the Office of Health Economics in *The Health Care Dilemma or 'Am I Kranken Doctor'?*, OHE, 1975.

Figure 1:
Proportion of total age group suffering from complaints in the 12 months to 31 March 1982

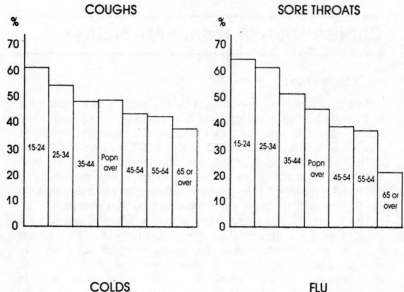

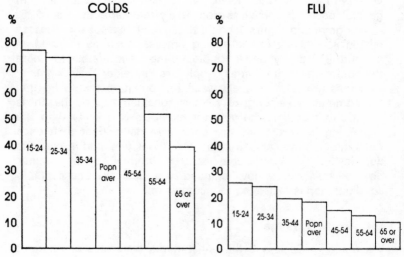

Source: The authors using data from the *Target Group Index* published by the British Market Research Bureau

Figure 1 (continued)

Proportion of total age group suffering from complaints in last 12 months

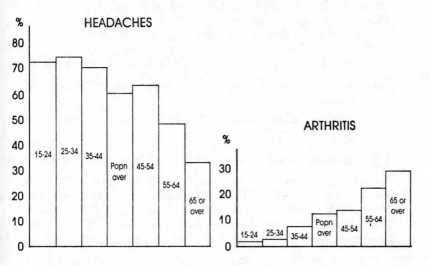

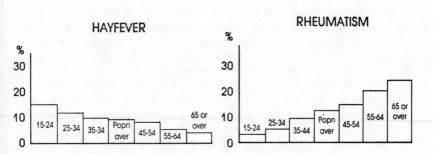

Source: The authors using data from the *Target Group Index*
published by the British Market Research Bureau

for ailments which doctors agree are the most appropriate for self-treatment; and, furthermore, that the medicines so purchased are the relevant treatments for the complaints. Not only are home medicines used sensibly—that is, the consumer does act responsibly in choosing between visiting a doctor and treating himself—but doctors claim that they are used successfully. Nine times out of 10, self-medication avoids the need to visit a doctor.

Dr R. V. M. Jones studied three sets of symptoms to discover:

(a) what proportions were taken to the doctor in the first instance;

(b) what proportions were treated with home medicines alone; and

(c) what proportions were treated first with home medicine.[1]

For indigestion, less than 7 per cent of the self-treated subsequently needed to visit the doctor; for coughs and colds, less than 9 per cent; and for diarrhoea and sickness, 34 per cent. Overall, only 11 per cent of self-treated cases were later presented to the doctor because self-medication had 'failed'. As Jones remarked:

'A "success-rate" of nearly 90 per cent for self-medication for coughs and colds, indigestion, diarrhoea and sickness emphasises the large and valuable part that self-medication plays in the day-to-day management of illness'.

(c) Advertising

Advertising of home medicines promotes better health because of the contribution it makes to health education. It is an efficient and reliable way of informing the public about the availability of medicines which they can take without prescription. Certainly, doctors, pharmacists and nurses are primary sources of professional advice about which medicines to purchase and when to use them. Formal health education, in schools and elsewhere, can also play an important role. Magazines, books and television provide considerable information, whilst relatives and friends are frequent sources of advice on health matters generally.

The purpose of advertising home medicines is either to remind existing users of the benefits of a product or to arouse the interest of potential new users sufficiently to persuade them to seek further information—from a professional adviser or by reading the information on the product package. It can also advise when

---

[1] R. V. M. Jones, 'Self-medication in a small community', *Journal of the Royal College of General Practitioners*, No. 26, 1976, p. 40.

an OTC product costs less than a prescription charge. The potential new user needs to acquire directions for use on dosage, frequency of administration, etc. Such information is found on the labels of all home medicines, complete with precautionary advice required under the terms of the product licence issued by the Department of Health.

Does advertising reflect these consumer requirements for information? Unfortunately, the data available on advertising expenditures, on market size by sales, and on market size by number of sufferers from a given complaint are not directly comparable. Nevertheless, several broad conclusions can be drawn and comparisons made.

Home medicines are not required by all consumers all the time. Despite this, they resemble other fast-moving, inexpensive consumer goods. Advertising information is not perused for days or weeks, as it may be for a high-priced, infrequently purchased good such as a car or a hi-fi set. The consumer desires a home medicine to give fast relief from his symptoms. Thus the advertising must be constant and extensive, and aimed at the fit population as well as the ill, since the former are potential customers and no method is available to detect how to advertise to them in advance of an ailment. Thus home medicine advertising must often appear obtrusive to the well, even though it is of immediate value to the sick.

Nevertheless, as Table 6 indicates, the industry does try to ensure an efficient minimisation of waste for certain categories of disease. Remedies for coughs, colds and 'flu, and for muscular and rheumatic conditions, are advertised in the months of the year when these ailments are likely to be prevalent for climatic reasons. Analgesics and travel pills are unfortunately treated as one in the advertising data, but there is a minimum below which advertising never falls (headaches are year-round phenomena). There are seasonal peaks in the winter months when analgesics are used by consumers for colds and 'flu and in the summer months when holidays increase the use of travel pills. Similarly, vitamin preparations are advertised least in the summer when climate can again be expected to boost general feelings of fitness. Advertising consequently varies according to the time of year.

Home medicine advertising is geared closely to the number of complainants, as Table 7 and Figure 2 show. This may seem at odds with the observation two paragraphs above that the fit have to be communicated with as well as the sick. To imagine, however, that the whole adult population would require identical expenditure on advertising, no matter the disease, would be to ignore

Table 6:
Advertising Expenditures on Home Medicines: By Month, 1982

(£'000)

	Jan.	Feb.	March	Apr.	May	June	July	Aug.	Sept.	Oct.	Nov.	Dec.
Oral hygiene	48·0	48·7	309·3	100·3	181·8	85·4	450·2	63·5	59·0	61·1	41·7	76·4
Cough remedies	2,147·1	845·5	22·3	–	0·1	1·0	0·2	–	13·4	472·6	1,141·5	1,603·4
Colds and 'flu	1,047·8	518·0	15·9	9·0	–	–	–	–	–	265·5	723·3	790·2
Analgesics, travel pills	1,448·7	1,245·1	780·5	988·7	367·6	612·7	733·6	1,061·6	1,175·8	942·7	939·8	621·4
Indigestion remedies	477·5	116·0	66·3	681·2	289·8	48·0	382·2	549·6	216·2	295·8	80·4	220·9
Muscular and rheumatism remedies	39·6	65·2	49·0	27·0	23·6	1·3	0·1	1·0	54·3	94·5	25·7	4·7
Vitamin preparations and tonics	1,034·6	566·9	332·5	263·5	178·7	184·2	144·2	217·3	288·6	1,149·4	520·0	249·0
Laxatives and salts	14·8	26·7	25·7	20·8	30·5	58·4	15·0	72·1	36·7	81·0	69·3	14·8

Source: MEAL, Quarterly Digest of Advertising Statistics.

a number of factors. As we have seen, rheumatism and arthritis are primarily diseases of the old. Thus advertising can be restricted (in relative terms) to the particular printed media or television viewing times to which the elderly are more exposed. This permits economies in advertising outlays.

Table 7:
Advertising Expenditure and Number of Complainants, 1982

Market	Advertising £'000	Nos. millions	Complaint
Analgesics	10,888	27	Headaches and migraine
Cough remedies	6,247	24	Coughs and colds
Indigestion remedies	3,424	14·1	Indigestion
Cold and 'flu remedies	3,370	7·9	'Flu
Muscular and rheum. remedies	386	5·4	Rheumatism and arthritis

Source: Target Group Index and MEAL.

Note: Data adjusted for comparability where necessary.

A third factor which is ignored by suggestions that advertising should be crudely linked to the size of the total adult population is an amalgam of the issues discussed above. Headaches are a year-round ailment and we would therefore expect (as indeed Table 6 substantiates) that expenditure on advertising analgesics would be relatively consistent throughout the year. Other things equal, such advertising expenditure and total complaints would both be higher (since 'complaints' indicate market size and hence are a proxy for the demand for advertising information). This is indeed so, as Figure 2 indicates.

Other variables, such as the degree of competition and innovation, are obviously not embraced in Figure 2. The data do support the view, however, that home medicine advertising has a distinct rationale, that advertisers are aware of this, and, like any profit-maximising businessmen, do not wish to spend resources in a wasteful fashion.

(d) Price Regulation of Home Medicines
Home medicines, like prescription medicines, are regulated or controlled in the entire marketing mix. The mix (or '4Ps', as

Figure 2:
Advertising expenditure and number of complainants by disease category, 1982

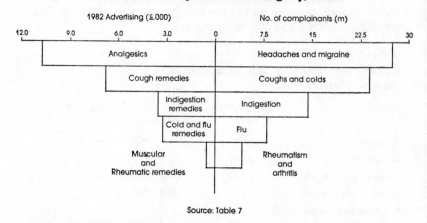

Source: Table 7

Professor E. J. McCarthy called it)[1] consists of price, place (or distribution channel), product, and promotion decisions.

Home medicines are one of the very few product groups on sale to the UK consumer whose prices are regulated. They are regulated in so far as home medicines have been judged exempt from the provisions of the Resale Prices Act of 1964, which prohibited resale price maintenance by individual manufacturers (that is, a manufacturer cannot stipulate a resale price to a retailer and, if the latter sells at a different price, penalise him by, for example, discontinuing supply). Pharmaceuticals are the only products to have been given such exemption in the 20 years since the Act was passed. The grounds for the exemption were that the fixed prices (and so guaranteed gross margins) were necessary to protect the wholesale and retail chemist whose skills and expertise were necessary for the protection of the public.

That the issues of the expertise of pharmacists and price competition should be linked in this way has already been criticised. There is no question that the pharmacist has a valuable role to play in community health care—not only in aiding choice and in providing professional advice about home medicines less well understood by patients, but also in assisting patients or customers to comply with manufacturers' recommendations.

---

[1] E. J. McCarthy, *Basic Marketing*, 2nd edn., Irwin, 1968.

(e) The Pharmacist's Role

The problem of non-compliant patients (those who do not take medicines in accordance with the instructions on the label or package) ranges from the trivial to the serious. Some forget to take the occasional tablet, or take rather too large a dosage. Others 'feel better' before a treatment has been completed, whilst others may 'feel worse'; both leave medicine unused. For the former, a relapse becomes more probable; for the latter, the initial side-effects or lack of a cure because of insufficiently prolonged medication may increase their long-term discomfort.

The non-compliance of consumers with manufacturers' instructions has been studied by a number of writers. Table 8 presents the results of a survey of such studies.

Overwhelmingly, the reasons for non-compliance stem from dissatisfaction with the treatment, either because of side-effects or because the patients are feeling worse after the medicine. Those reasons were mentioned in 30 out of 78 studies in which consumers of medicine gave some explanation for non-compliance. By contrast, only five out of the 78 studies referred to confusion as a cause of non-compliance, and only four to 'financial need'. A low price may be attractive but price *per se* does not appear to be of major importance, to consumers at least, as a deterrent to health and consumption.

By inference, Table 8 also suggests that the advertising, packaging and labelling methods and the written instructions provided by manufacturers are, by and large, of a helpful, straightforward

Table 8:
Reasons Given by Patients for Non-Compliance with Instructions on Medicines

Number of Studies Mentioning:

Side-effects	15
Dissatisfaction (feeling worse)	15
Feeling better	12
Forgetting	7
Confusion	5
Financial need	4
Others	20

Source: Brian Haynes, Wayne Taylor and David Sackett, *Compliance in Health Care*, Johns Hopkins Press, 1977.

kind. The 42 instances where patients voluntarily did not comply raise two issues. Was the non-compliance intelligent and sensible? Was the non-compliance due to the selection of an inappropriate medicine?

As for the first issue, there are clearly times when voluntary non-compliance is appropriate and the consumer will know his state of health better than an outsider. The more minor the ailment, the more likely this is to be true (short-lived headaches, for example). Where the medicine is curative rather than symptom-relieving, however, there is scope for outside advice of a kind flexible enough for the individual requirements of the consumer. There is thus considerable scope for verbal dialogue between pharmacist and customer in those instances where labelling and packaging information cannot be wholly comprehensive. This would enhance the pharmacist's role in health care and increase the efficiency of the system for delivering health care. Of course, such a dialogue would have to be initiated; here again, media advertising could perform a vital role in motivating consumers to consult their pharmacist.

The second issue prompts the following question: Was the inappropriate medicine selected because the range of choice facing the consumer was so wide as to 'confuse' him in his choice of a product (although not in his *use* of it)—and hence to make him 'dissatisfied' or suffer 'side-effects'? Again, it seems that there is not only a role for advertising to inform consumers of the range of choice, but that there is a unqiue and valuable role for the pharmacist also. The customer will benefit from a wide range of medicines only if he takes enough trouble to choose one which is appropriate to his requirements. If this demands more time or expertise than he has available, the pharmacist can assist him.

This analysis, based on American experience, suggests that the assistance pharmacies give to consumers is important in the USA, and that it accompanies price competition at the retail stage. This conclusion is consistent with pharmaceutical experience in other countries, and with other types of professional retailing in Britain. For example, in other countries where pharmacists do compete on price—not only for home medicines but also for prescription medicines—the pharmacy continues to exist side-by-side with such outlets as neighbouring supermarkets. And the pharmacist maintains his service and advice.

(f) Should Price Regulation be Retained?

Almost identical claims about preserving professional services were made in the UK by book publishers. In 1962, the Net Book Agreement (whereby publishers collectively enforce resale price maintenance) was permitted to stand despite its *prima facie* breach of the 1956 Restrictive Trade Practices Act.[1] The Net Book Agreement was allowed to continue because, claimed the publishers, the public would be deprived of the services of the specialist bookseller if price competition were permitted in book retailing—an argument similar to that for RPM in home medicines. Yet the same claim could have been made for the sale of musical records and cassettes: namely, that the specialist record shop would be unable to compete with lower-price, general retailers. The record manufacturers, however, never had an agreement as strong or as visible as that of the publishers and price competition has obtained in record retailing for over three decades with no apparent deterioration in the service given by specialist retailers.

The pharmaceutical profession and several spokesmen for manufacturers of home medicines argue that the price collusion permitted by law is necessary to ensure that the pharmacist can survive to provide his services. As outside observers, however, the authors of this *Research Monograph* are not convinced that the pharmacy profession is unique and different from professions such as law, accountancy, optometry and opticians' services where price competition is permitted in Britain at the retail level, and where standards of service tend to be maintained and consumer prices reduced. It is at least possible that the lack of price competition when advertising is reduced results in somnolence such that pharmacists in general are *not* spurred to provide the services to the consumer which only they are able to supply.

(g) Rivalry by Distribution Channels

Competition in home medicines is regulated not only by price but also by location.[2] There is, in other words, legislation which controls distribution channels. The enabling legislation for such regulation was the Medicines Act of 1968. Since it was passed, however, a variety of new or revised statutory instruments have come into being. For example, the General Sale List (GSL), implemented in January 1981, revoked four previous such lists which had been operating since 1978 (all consequential on the

---

[1] The 1956 Act banned collective agreements by manufacturers to enforce resale price maintenance; the 1964 Resale Prices Act dealt with individual manufacturers.

[2] That is, place, the second of McCarthy's '4Ps' of the marketing mix.

Table 9:
Sales Turnover of Pharmacies and Drug Stores:
UK, year to October, 1979 and 1980

Percentages of Total Turnover	Year to October 1979	1980
Pharmacies	80	80
Drug Stores	20	20

Percentages of Turnover of Nine Proprietary Medicine Categories		
Pharmacies	91	92
Drug Stores	9	8

Source: Nielsen Researcher, 1981.

1968 Medicines Act). The List details products 'which in the opinion of the Ministers can with reasonable safety be sold or supplied otherwise than by or under the supervision of a pharmacist' (General Sale List, p. 3). There are 75 pages detailing such products in the 1981 GSL. Another statutory instrument (The Medicines Sale or Supply Regulations), which also followed the 1968 Act, came into force in 1980. This provides the retail pharmacist with still more protection. It prohibits outlets other than pharmacies from selling analgesics such as aspirin in packs above a certain size, and even pharmacies are exempt only when the qualified pharmacist is on the premises.[1]

The benefits to the retail pharmacist of this legislation are considerable, as Tables 9 and 10 indicate. There the sales of retail pharmacies are compared with a newly-emerging type of retailer— the specialist home medicine and general drug store (Superdrug, for example) which does not employ a qualified pharmacist. The Tables compare the positions of the two types of retailer before and after the relevant Sale or Supply statutory instrument was enforced.

Drug stores operating without a pharmacist have been able to hold their own, with 20 per cent of total (that is, pharmacy plus drug store) sales, despite the legislation. Pharmacies, on the other

---

[1] Thus the consumer is now placed in the faintly ridiculous position of being unable to buy a bottle of 100 aspirin tablets from a supermarket, but only a relatively more costly pack of, say, 10. Furthermore, he cannot even purchase a bottle of 100 such tablets from a retail pharmacist if the pharmacist is off the premises, as he often is—indeed, daily at lunch-time—in single-pharmacist stores. Yet sales constantly take place while the pharmacist is in another part of the same building!

Table 10:
Indices of Rates of Sale* of Proprietary Medicines:
Year to October, 1979 and 1980

Product Categories	Retail Pharmacies	Drug Stores 1979	1980
Indigestion tablets	100*	111*	117*
Oral analgesic tablets and powders	100	110	58
Stomach upset remedies	100	154	176
Cough liquids	100	26	27
Cough/cold pastilles and lozenges	100	79	87
Nerve tonic and multi-vitamins	100	64	66
Oral lesion preparations	100	58	40
Sprays and drops	100	36	36
Vapour rubs	100	81	92

Note: This implies that, given an index of 100 for pharmacies, drug store sales of indigestion tablets, for example, rose 11 per cent more than pharmacy sales in 1979 and 17 per cent more in 1980.

Source: Nielsen Researcher, 1981.

hand, have increased their market share (from 91 to 92 per cent) exclusively in proprietary medicines where they are protected from competition on both price and location.

Table 9 is hardly significant statistically. Table 10, however, examines the medicines in more detail and shows that the strength of retail pharmacies in 1980 was entirely due to the legislation limiting the sizes and brands of proprietary medicines available in other outlets. The data given in Table 10 highlight the spectacular fall in oral analgesic sales (where the legislation was most restrictive). According to the *Nielsen Researcher*, 'this one product category accounted *for the whole increase* shown by pharmacists' in the nine proprietary medicine categories of Table 9 (emphasis added). In other (unprotected) medicine categories, pharmacies have lost ground as consumers have steadily shifted their purchases to more preferred outlets.

Regulation of home medicines thus protects the retail pharmacist from competition in terms of both price and place. Consumers are prevented from purchasing products at prices or locations they would presumably prefer.

(h) Product Rivalry

The legislation has been ambivalent about the third of McCarthy's 'Ps', *product* competition. The Medicines Act of 1968 affected both the prescription and the home medicine industries. The licensing procedures it introduced before a new product can be marketed have proven to be cumbersome, time-consuming and costly in both industries.[1] As a consequence, innovations have been fewer in number, and a new product takes longer than might otherwise be necessary to reach the market-place. The Government is aware of the problem, however, and has shortened the process by means of a 'fast track' for uncomplicated applications. This change is especially relevant to the home medicine industry where many new products are representations or re-combinations of tried and tested preparations already available.[2]

The other source of new products for the home medicine industry is the official re-classification for pharmacy sale of drugs which are currently prescription-only. The regulatory trend is to encourage this movement—in contrast with the 1950s when Oblivon (the first of the tranquillisers, discovered and marketed in the UK by Aspro-Nicholas) was transferred in the reverse direction from non-prescription to prescription-only.

In the United States, the Commissioner of the Food and Drug Administration, Dr Arthur Hull Mayer, has argued that people

'throughout the world are taking greater charge of their own health maintenance and care . . . because they are personally motivated by feelings of their own competence and a desire for self-sufficiency'.[3]

One major ingredient has now made the switch from prescription-only to pharmacy sale without prescription in the USA. The product, 0·5 per cent hydrocortisone, has a long track-record for safety and efficacy in dermatological uses. This change has meant that hydrocortisone products for the relief of minor skin ailments are now readily available to the consumer. Competition among manufacturers has increased which is benefiting the consumer in the form of lower prices and/or more acceptable presentations of products.

---

[1] K. Hartley and A. Maynard, 'The Regulation of the UK Pharmaceutical Industry: A Cost-Benefit Analysis', *Managerial and Decision Economics*, Vol. 3, 1982; W. D. Reekie, 'Legislative Change and Industrial Performance: A Case Study', *Scottish Journal of Political Economy*, 1980.

[2] The 'fast track' is known formally as the Abridged Product Licence Application procedure which requires less information from an applicant company about a product's action—and hence less monitoring of performance by the firm and less screening of those results by the DHSS.

[3] Cited in the *PAGB Annual Report*, 1981-82.

The current politico-economic climate is favourable to this type of switch. Not only are more prescription-only products becoming mature and well-understood by both prescribers and patients; the cost of the NHS as a whole has increased by 50 per cent in real terms since it was founded—from 4 per cent of GNP in 1949, 4·28 in 1966, 5·19 in 1974, to nearly 6·2 per cent in 1984 (the comparable figures for the USA are 4·4 per cent in 1954 and 10·5 per cent in 1982). There is thus considerable pressure to contain what is sometimes called the 'health-care cost explosion'. Moreover, the experience of the UK and US is in no way unique; governments throughout the world are concerned about spiralling health-care expenditure and are seeking ways to contain costs and make the most efficient use of the resources available.

'Responsible self-medication' to encourage NHS economy

One way of containing costs is to encourage self-medication. Responsible self-medication in the treatment of minor ailments is increasingly seen to have a major role to play in ensuring that resources are used to their best advantage. It is not that self-medication offers a substitute for the care of doctors; rather, the proper use of home medicines by the public in the self-treatment of minor ailments complements medical consultation, and as such can relieve pressure on primary-care services and release significant resources for the treatment of conditions which demand professional attention. That the capacity for self-care represents a valuable resource was recognised by the Royal Commission on the National Health Service which reported in 1979 that

'intelligent self-medication and care can undoubtedly reduce demands on health services, and it is essential that society accepts the need for appropriate self-care'.[1]

And on 27 July 1979, *Hansard* recorded the then Minister of State for Health agreeing that

'all concerned [should be] aware of the proper place of drugs in treatment and their limitations, and [there should be] a commonsense self-reliance in the management and avoidance of minor disorders'.

A number of products have now been removed from the prescription-only list arising out of the Medicines Act. They include an anti-diarrhoeal (Loperamide) and a big-selling, non-steroidal, anti-inflammatory analgesic (ibuprofen) which was

---

[1] *Report of the Royal Commission on the National Health Service* (Chairman: Sir Alec Merrison), Cmnd. 7615, HMSO, July 1979.

discovered by Boots Limited and promoted to doctors under the brand name Brufen—and now to the general public as Nurofen. This re-classification is as major a breakthrough in the UK as 0·5 per cent hydrocortisone was in the USA. In 1982, according to the Office of Health Economics, 60 million arthritis patients a year worldwide were being treated with Brufen.

Table 11 suggests the scope for savings to the NHS on some products if more re-classification of drugs and/or more self-medication were encouraged. It shows many of the principal areas where self-medication is already possible, or where it could be regarded as already existing given the prevalence of 'repeat prescriptions' (hypnotics and sedatives, for example). It also illustrates the potential benefit to the NHS of enhanced competition in home medicine products: in 1982 prices, £324 million of resources used in the NHS could have been re-directed to other areas of health care—and this figure is probably conservative because it takes no account of the associated savings in the consultation time of doctors.

Table 11:
Numbers and Cost of Prescriptions: UK, 1982

	Prescriptions (million)	Ingredient cost* per prescription (£)	Total cost* (£million)
Expectorants and cough suppressants	14·4	1·21	17·42
Minor analgesics	21·0	1·79	37·59
Vitamins	4·4	1·71	7·52
Anti-inflammatory preparations for rheumatism (e.g. ibuprofen)	18·9	6·59	124·55
Preparations for topical use in skin conditions (e.g. 0·5% hydrocortisone)	22·8	2·11	48·11
Anti-diarrhoeals	3·0	2·20	6·60
Laxatives	5·0	1·67	8·35
Antacids (indigestion remedies)	6·8	1·99	13·53
Sleeping tablets (hypnotics)	16·9	1·66	28·05
Sedatives and tranquillisers (e.g. Valium)	21·4	1·49	31·89
			£323·61

*Note: 'Ingredient cost' is the price paid to the manufacturer. 'Total cost' includes dispensing fee, on-cost and pharmacists' container allowances.

Source: Office of Health Economics, Compendium of Health Statistics, 1984.

Such a shift to self-medication, of course, would only be possible with a judicious use of McCarthy's fourth 'p', *promotion*, and the provision of information for patients. Certainly, for many diseases, the diagnosis, the selection of therapy and the monitoring of progress are the exclusive preserves of the doctor. But for other conditions, such as maintenance therapy or the management of symptoms of chronic ailments—arthritis or insomnia, perhaps—there may be a larger role for the patient in decision-making (within controlled limits) about when to alter dosages or the frequency of his prescribed regimen so that he does not necessarily have to consult the doctor on each occasion. The pharmacist, with his unique blend of professional skills and public accessibility, can clearly have a crucial advisory role to play here.[1]

(i) Ownership Regulation

The preferences of consumers are shifting (in relative terms) towards purchasing from pharmacy chains rather than independent retailers. This development is similar to the revolution which occurred in grocery retailing in the 1950s and early-1960s. In some countries, however, consumers' wishes cannot be expressed in this way. In Canada, West Germany and South Africa, for example, a pharmacy must be owned by a pharmacist, and this requirement precludes the development of multiple chains. Nonetheless, in Canada a so-called 'grandfather clause' in the rules enables chains such as Boots to purchase existing pharmacies on the retirement of an owner. In South Africa, manufacturers can provide loans to individuals to set up their own pharmacies. The loans are linked to promotional and other assistance. The relationship is similar to the voluntary groups and chains which exist in food retailing. However, common ownership is prohibited and, on the death or retirement of the owner, a pharmacy must be sold to another pharmacist within six months. Once again, rules ostensibly to protect the public deprive consumers of the kind of OTC provision of medicines they might prefer—and which, in countries such as the UK and USA, they have already shown they do prefer.

---

[1] In addition to the shift to OTC sales of the products mentioned above, the following ingredients have recently been moved from prescription-only sale: 0·5 per cent hydrocortisone (New Zealand, New South Wales); 1·0 per cent hydrocortisone (Sweden); nitrazepam and temazepam (New South Wales); clotrimazole, econazole nitrate, isoconazole nitrate and miconazole nitrate (France); and tioconazole (USA). (This information was supplied to the authors by Professor Michael Cooper.)

Only consumers can determine the mix of price, product, place, promotion and ownership service they prefer. It is a false (and arrogant) assumption that regulators can do it for them.

APPENDIX TO SECTION THREE

The NHS Restricted List: A Topical Comment

The above discussion is particularly pertinent in the light of recent developments in the ethical (prescription-only) market. Mr Norman Fowler, Secretary of State for Health and Social Services recently announced his intention to restrict the number of drugs available under the NHS. He informed the House of Commons in February 1985[1] that there would be a 'black list', 31 pages long, of drugs which doctors would no longer be able to prescribe under the NHS—although they could continue to do so if the patient paid the full price. For example, no Roche tranquilliser or hypnotic (such as Valium or Mogadon) is on the 'white' permissible list. The cough syrup Benylin will also be prohibited. According to the *Financial Times*, 'this will probably mean the loss of hundreds of jobs' at Roche's operations in the United Kingdom.

The ethical industry, including firms such as Roche, has reacted sharply to this statement of intent by running a large and costly advertising campaign in the British press. In essence, it has argued that a research-based industry is under attack and that the attempt to control government costs by banning certain drugs will be counter-productive in the long run: firms denied revenue will cease to conduct research into new medicines.

The attack by government on the cost of ethical drugs could have been predicted by any student of monopsony.[2] A monopsonist will attempt to obtain the best terms of exchange or of trade in his favour. In this instance, the monopsonistic NHS has calculated that a reduction in the choice of products available to its customers is an acceptable price to be paid for reducing the cost to government of prescription drugs. The NHS—and its spokesman, the Secretary of State for Health and Social Services— can never represent the diverse interests of doctors, pharmacists

---

[1] *Financial Times*, 22 February 1985.

[2] Monopsony is a technical term meaning 'a single buyer', just as monopoly means a single seller.

and, most important of all, patients. Only individuals, acting for themselves, can know the unique circumstances of their therapeutic needs. Only individuals can take optimal decisions. It is beyond the bounds of any rules of probability that the Secretary of State could produce a unique list of medicines which would simultaneously accommodate a multitude of illnesses and reactions, medical diagnoses and pharmaceutical skills.

It is at least arguable that, rather than removing a doctor's freedom to prescribe, government should further enlarge the pharmacist's freedom to dispense for self-medication. Simultaneously, this would accomplish Mr Fowler's desire to save on NHS spending, would not deny corporations revenue required to fund research and development, and would harness more effectively the pharmacist's professional skills.

The argument that the 'poor would suffer' because they could not afford to pay for the drugs released from prescription-only categories can be turned neatly aside. First, as we have seen, price does not deter most people from purchasing OTC medicines. Secondly, the provision of any item (including a health-care component such as a medicine) through private or state insurance should be carried out only if the two main reasons for insurance exist: that is, the event insured against must be catastrophic and unlikely. These two conditions do not hold for medicines, ethical or OTC. Medicines are bought and consumed frequently and their unit cost is low.[1] Certainly, the chronic sick on constant medication who are also indigent might be unable to meet their medical bills. But they are a small proportion of the total community and their needs can be met through some form of social security which caters exclusively for them and not through a panoply of controls governing the entire pharmacy and medical professions, the ethical and OTC manufacturing industries and, by implication, each and every member of the British population.

---

[1] For 1983, the Office of Health Economics has calculated that the average *total* (i.e. including distributors' margins, etc) prescription cost in the UK was £4.16.

51

FOUR

Conclusions

Economic competition in price, product, place, promotion and ownership has a valuable and essential role to play in the home medicine industry.

1. Home medicines are used responsibly by consumers and their use releases resources for more serious ailments.
2. Advertising can reduce the burden placed on the doctor by bringing to the patient's attention home medicines suitable for his condition.
3. Home medicines are heavily promoted because the promotion must reach the healthy as well as the sick so that the latter have at hand a store of information about products.
4. Nevertheless, firms attempt to minimise unnecessary advertising by targeting their messages to high-risk social groups and during high-risk times of the year.
5. Regulation of the industry is declining in some respects and increasing in others.
6. It is declining as more and more medicines which were formerly prescription-only are removed to the General Sale List or, less freely, to pharmacy-only sale. These medicines have been tried and tested over the years and shown to be efficacious and relatively safe. This trend will continue as more and more of the drugs discovered in the prescription medicine industry during the 1950s and 1960s become mature, and as patients become more self-reliant and willing to undertake the responsibility of self-cures.
7. Such a trend will enlarge the volume of promotion required to inform patients about new products and about the re-combinations and representations of existing agents which have been the main source of innovation in recent years.
8. In contrast, resale price maintenance continues to prevent price competition, and competition among products has been

increasingly hampered by the regulatory provisions of the Medicines Act. Firms have thus left the industry, further reducing competition of all kinds. Competition by place of sale is now more restricted than ever, even for medicines (such as aspirin) which have been distributed safely and widely for half a century. And certain products are no longer allowed to be publicly advertised. These restrictions have harmed the consumer, the producer, and those specialist and other retailers of drugs who operate without a pharmacist on the premises.

9. The industry has considerable growth potential as more and more products are released from the prescription-only category. This, in turn, will enhance the potential role of the retail pharmacist as a health-care professional. His task of assisting the individual consumer to select the precise medicine for his needs will increase, thereby simultaneously reducing the burden of the National Health Service to the taxpayer.

10. Experience from overseas suggests that pharmacies can exist without the benefit of 'fair trade' laws or RPM. Given the potential increase in the number of new OTC products, the position of the professional pharmacist appears secure. Furthermore, it would be both more economically efficient and more professionally satisfying to the pharmacist if he were to become a purveyor of advice to consumers about products rather than merely a 'pill-counter' and 'shelf-filler'. If the consumer is free to choose which type of retail outlet he patronises, there is no reason to believe he will be so foolish as to avoid the pharmacy with its unique package of products and professional advice.

How far proposals to deregulate the OTC industry can be carried is still a debatable issue. Whether or not the benefits of wider distribution, a broader range of product choice and lower prices would be offset by irresponsible consumption cannot be wholly determined. Seen against the contemporary OTC industry in other countries, however, it would appear that considerable deregulation could be undertaken to the substantial advantage of the British economy and British consumers in general. In particular, we would recommend:

(a) that resale price maintenance in pharmaceuticals be forbidden as a restrictive trade practice;

(b) that the position before the Medicines Act of 1968 be

restored so that more medicines can be sold in non-pharmacy outlets and advertised to consumers;

and

(c) that the speed with which medicines are being switched from prescription-only to OTC sale be accelerated.

Some recent IEA publications

economics affairs

A quarterly journal of economic analysis and commentary, published by Longman Group Limited in association with the Institute of Economic Affairs

Editor: Arthur Seldon

Economic Affairs is topical, readable and provocative. It provides economists with a forum to discuss recent, current and impending developments, allowing them to respond quickly to new trends and events.

In concise, non-technical language authors challenge accepted wisdom. Using both micro- and macro-economic methods, they shed light on traditional economic subjects and extend the use of economic analysis to a host of new occupations, services, products and industries.

Economic Affairs is read in 50 countries, by economists, government officials, businessmen, labour leaders, academics, teachers and students who need to keep up-to-date with current thinking.

Since 1980, **Economic Affairs** has published the work of over 250 authors from the UK and overseas, including:

Norman Barry – Michael Beenstock – Roy Batchelor – Mark Blaug – Alan Budd – Karl Brunner – John Burton – Frank Chapple – Anthony Christopher – Tim Congdon – Stanley Dennison – Walter Eltis – Edgar Feige – Herbert Giersch – David Green – Jo Grimond – Ralph Harris – F. A. Hayek – David Henderson – Sir Geoffrey Howe – Richard Jackman – Israel Kirzner – David Laidler – Stephen Littlechild – Allan Meltzer – Patrick Minford – Mancur Olson – David Owen – Kristian Palda–Alan Peacock– Lord Robbins – Colin Robinson – Anna Schwartz – Ljubo Sirc – Gordon Tullock – Roland Vaubel – E. G. West – Geoffrey Wood – Basil Yamey.

Economic Affairs   ISSN 0265-0665
published quarterly, in October, January, April and July.

For subscription details, please write to:
LONGMAN GROUP LTD.
Subscriptions Department (Journals),
Fourth Avenue, Harlow, Essex CM19 5AA, England.